# Natural Remedies for Insomnia

*Sleep Better with Holistic Nighttime Solutions*

**Nora Cobbs A.**

# Table of contents

# Introduction

Sleep is often referred to as the foundation of our well-being. Yet, for many, restful nights feel out of reach, a struggle that starts the moment their head hits the pillow. Insomnia can turn those quiet hours into a battleground of tossing, turning, and staring at the clock, hoping for sleep that never comes. But what if, instead of reaching for the same old quick fixes or prescription solutions, you had access to something more natural, gentle, and restorative?

Insomnia isn't just about sleepless nights. It's about the tiredness that seeps into every part of life—the foggy mornings, the inability to concentrate at work, the irritability in personal relationships, and the endless chase for energy that coffee and stimulants can't quite provide. When we can't sleep, everything feels out of balance, and the constant fatigue often leads us to feel disconnected from ourselves and the world around us.

The good news? You don't have to settle for this cycle. While modern medicine often points us toward pills and quick fixes, natural remedies provide a deeper, longer-lasting solution to one of life's most frustrating problems. These methods work with your body's natural rhythms rather than against them, offering a path to healing that doesn't just cover up the symptoms but addresses the root causes of your sleepless nights.

In this book, you'll discover a treasure trove of holistic strategies that tap into the body's innate ability to find peace and balance. From calming foods and herbal teas to soothing bedtime routines and mindfulness techniques, these tools offer more than just sleep—they offer the kind of rest that nourishes the soul. This is not about popping a pill and hoping for the best. This is about building a sustainable, long-term relationship with sleep that allows you to wake up every day feeling rejuvenated, not just rested.

What you will find ahead isn't a one-size-fits-all approach but rather a collection of practices that can be tailored to your individual needs. With each page, you'll explore new ways to improve your sleep, guided by natural remedies that work in harmony with your body. By the end, you'll not only be equipped with the knowledge to conquer insomnia but also to reclaim the vibrant, energized life that sleep-deprivation has taken from you.

Welcome to a journey where sleep doesn't have to be a distant dream—it can become a natural part of your everyday routine, leaving you ready to embrace life fully, starting from tonight.

# Chapter 1: Understanding Insomnia

## Types of Insomnia: Acute vs. Chronic

Insomnia can take on different forms, depending on its duration and intensity. **Acute insomnia** is typically short-term and often tied to specific life events or stressors. A sudden work deadline, a major shift in routine, or emotional distress can trigger episodes of sleeplessness. These periods can last a few nights to a few weeks and usually resolve once the underlying issue is addressed. While disruptive, acute insomnia tends to be temporary and subsides when the cause is removed, allowing individuals to return to a normal sleep pattern.

In contrast, **chronic insomnia** is much more persistent, lasting for months or even years. It becomes a regular part of life, with sufferers experiencing sleepless nights at least three times a week over an extended period. Chronic insomnia doesn't simply fade away when stress or routine changes; it becomes a constant struggle, leading to exhaustion, irritability, and cognitive impairment. Those facing chronic insomnia often feel trapped in a cycle of sleep deprivation that no amount of routine tweaking or temporary fixes seem to resolve.

## Common Causes of Insomnia

There's no single cause for insomnia. Instead, it can arise from a combination of factors, both physical and psychological. One of the most prevalent causes is **stress**. Whether related to personal life, work, or broader societal pressures, stress keeps the mind racing when it should be winding down. Worries about the future, relationships, or looming deadlines can create an overactive mind that resists rest.

**Diet** also plays a crucial role. Consuming stimulants like caffeine or high-sugar foods, especially in the hours leading up to bedtime, can interfere with the body's ability to relax. Late-night meals, particularly those high in fat or spice, can cause discomfort, indigestion, or acid reflux, all of which make it harder to fall asleep.

Alcohol, while often thought of as a relaxant, can disrupt sleep cycles and prevent deep, restorative rest.

**Lifestyle factors** also contribute significantly. People who have irregular sleep schedules, such as those who stay up late on weekends but rise early during the week, often struggle to maintain a consistent sleep-wake cycle. Similarly, lack of physical activity during the day can leave the body insufficiently tired at night. Additionally, the increasing reliance on screens, particularly in the evening, is a major issue. The blue light emitted from smartphones, tablets, and televisions tricks the brain into staying alert by mimicking daylight, thereby delaying the production of melatonin, the hormone responsible for regulating sleep.

## How Lack of Sleep Affects the Body and Mind

The effects of sleep deprivation ripple throughout every aspect of life. Physically, **lack of sleep** weakens the immune system, making it harder to fight off infections. It increases the risk of chronic conditions like heart disease, diabetes, and obesity. When sleep is consistently compromised, the body's ability to regulate hormones like insulin and cortisol is disrupted, leading to heightened inflammation and stress levels.

Mentally, the impact of poor sleep is just as profound. Cognitive function is significantly impaired, making it harder to focus, solve problems, or process information. Memory can become unreliable, with short-term recall in particular being affected. Emotional regulation also suffers, with mood swings, irritability, and feelings of anxiety or depression becoming more common. Over time, chronic sleep deprivation can even alter brain chemistry, making it harder to manage stress and maintain a positive outlook.

## When to Seek Medical Advice

While occasional sleeplessness is a common experience, there are times when professional help is necessary. If insomnia persists for more than a few weeks, or if it begins to interfere with daily functioning—such as affecting work, relationships, or overall quality of life—it's important to consult a healthcare provider.

Persistent fatigue, mood changes, or an inability to focus might signal underlying issues that require medical attention. Additionally, if lifestyle changes, natural remedies, or sleep hygiene improvements fail to bring relief, a doctor can help assess whether there are more serious conditions, like sleep apnea, restless leg syndrome, or depression, that need to be addressed.

# Chapter 2: The Role of Diet in Better Sleep

## Foods That Promote Sleep

The foods you consume throughout the day, especially in the evening, can significantly impact your ability to fall asleep and stay asleep. Certain foods are rich in nutrients that promote relaxation and improve sleep quality. **Magnesium-rich foods** are particularly beneficial, as magnesium is known to regulate melatonin levels and relax muscles, easing the body into sleep. Foods like spinach, almonds, bananas, and avocados are great sources of magnesium. Incorporating these into your evening meal can help calm the nervous system and prepare the body for restful sleep.

Another category of sleep-enhancing foods includes those high in **tryptophan**, an amino acid that helps the body produce serotonin and melatonin. Turkey, chicken, oats, and eggs are good options that can be easily added to dinner. Additionally, foods like **kiwi** and **cherries** are naturally high in melatonin, the hormone responsible for regulating sleep-wake cycles. Having a small portion of these fruits in the evening can be a natural way to signal to the body that it's time to wind down.

For those who enjoy a calming ritual before bed, **herbal teas** can be incredibly soothing. Chamomile tea, in particular, has been used for centuries to aid relaxation and improve sleep quality. It contains antioxidants like apigenin, which bind to receptors in the brain that may reduce anxiety and initiate sleep. Other beneficial teas include **peppermint**, which helps with digestion and can prevent discomfort that may keep you awake, and **lavender**, known for its calming properties that ease tension and stress.

## Foods to Avoid

Just as some foods promote sleep, others can seriously interfere with your ability to drift off. **Caffeine** is the most obvious culprit. Found in coffee, certain teas, chocolate, and many energy drinks, caffeine is a powerful stimulant that can stay in your system for hours. Drinking caffeine in the afternoon or evening can prevent you from falling asleep by blocking the chemicals in your brain that help induce sleepiness. It's important to keep caffeine consumption to the early part of the day and opt for non-caffeinated beverages in the evening.

**Sugar** is another substance to watch out for. While it may provide a quick energy boost, consuming sugar before bed can lead to blood sugar spikes and crashes, which may disturb your sleep cycles. Desserts, sugary snacks, and processed foods can leave you feeling restless and jittery, making it harder for your body to settle into sleep.

**Heavy meals**, particularly those high in fat or spice, should also be avoided close to bedtime. Eating large portions can make your body work overtime to digest the food, leading to discomfort, indigestion, and even acid reflux. This physical discomfort can interfere with your ability to relax, making it difficult to fall asleep. Aim to have your last meal at least two to three hours before bedtime, and keep it light to avoid digestive disruptions.

## Sleep-Inducing Beverages and Herbal Infusions

In addition to solid foods, there are several beverages and infusions that can encourage sleep. **Warm milk** is a classic remedy that has been passed down through generations. Milk contains both tryptophan and calcium, which work together to produce melatonin. The warmth of the milk also has a naturally calming effect, making it a comforting option for many before bed.

If you prefer non-dairy alternatives, **herbal infusions** like **chamomile**, **valerian root**, and **lemon balm** teas are excellent choices. These herbs are known for their calming effects and ability to reduce stress and anxiety, helping you unwind from the day's pressures. **Tart cherry juice** is another option, as cherries are one of the few natural sources of melatonin. Drinking a small glass of tart cherry juice before bed can help enhance sleep quality and duration.

**Golden milk**, made from a blend of turmeric, milk (or a non-dairy alternative), and a touch of honey, is another beverage gaining popularity for its sleep-inducing properties. Turmeric contains curcumin, which has anti-inflammatory effects and may help reduce stress and improve relaxation. Adding a pinch of cinnamon or ginger can further enhance its calming effects.

Incorporating these sleep-promoting foods and beverages into your evening routine can make a significant difference in your ability to fall asleep naturally and stay asleep throughout the night. Small changes in your diet can go a long way in improving overall sleep quality.

# Chapter 3: Creating a Sleep-Inducing Environment

## Importance of a Restful Bedroom

Creating an environment that fosters rest is essential for a good night's sleep, and the setup of your bedroom plays a significant role in determining the quality of your rest. **Lighting** is one of the most critical elements to consider. Exposure to artificial light, particularly blue light from screens, can interfere with your body's natural sleep-wake cycle. The hormone melatonin, which signals to your body that it's time to sleep, is suppressed by exposure to light. To promote better sleep, it's essential to dim the lights in the evening and eliminate or reduce light sources in your bedroom. Consider using blackout curtains to block out streetlights or early morning sunlight. Dimmable bedside lamps or low-wattage bulbs can also help transition your body from wakefulness to relaxation in the evening.

**Noise** is another factor that can make or break your sleep environment. While some people may prefer complete silence, others find a certain amount of ambient noise comforting. Either way, disruptive noises, such as traffic, barking dogs, or even the hum of appliances, can prevent you from falling asleep or cause you to wake up in the middle of the night. To counteract this, consider using a white noise machine or a fan to drown out disruptive sounds. Earplugs are also an effective, low-cost option to block out unwanted noise, providing a peaceful and quiet space for rest.

The **temperature** of your room is just as important as lighting and noise. The body naturally cools down as it prepares for sleep, so keeping your bedroom at a cool, comfortable temperature—typically between 60 to 67 degrees Fahrenheit—can help signal to your body that it's time to rest. A room that is too hot or too cold can disrupt your sleep, causing you to wake up frequently or struggle to fall asleep in the first place. Bedding choices, which we'll explore next, can also influence how well your body regulates temperature during the night.

## Sleep-Friendly Bedding and Pillows

The comfort of your **bedding and pillows** is a foundational part of ensuring a restful night. The goal is to create a cocoon of comfort that allows your body to fully relax and sink into sleep. Choosing the right materials for your bedding is essential, as it directly impacts how your body regulates temperature and comfort throughout the night. Natural, breathable fabrics such as cotton, linen, or bamboo are ideal, as they help wick away moisture and allow for airflow. This prevents overheating, which is a common cause of restless sleep.

When it comes to your **pillow**, it's important to find one that provides the right support for your preferred sleeping position. A pillow that is too flat or too thick can strain your neck and shoulders, leading to discomfort that might cause you to toss and turn during the night. For side sleepers, a thicker pillow can help align the neck and spine, while back sleepers generally benefit from a medium-firm pillow that supports the natural curvature of the neck. Stomach sleepers, on the other hand, may require a thinner pillow to prevent neck strain. Memory foam pillows or those made with natural latex offer a combination of softness and support, molding to the shape of your head and neck to promote proper alignment.

Your mattress is equally important in promoting restful sleep. A mattress that is too soft may cause your body to sink, leading to misalignment of the spine, while a mattress that is too firm can create pressure points, making it hard to stay comfortable throughout the night. It's important to choose a mattress that supports your body's needs, taking into account factors like your weight, sleeping position, and any physical ailments, such as back pain. Consider rotating your mattress regularly or using a mattress topper for additional comfort and support.

## Using Scents and Essential Oils

**Aromatherapy** can be a powerful tool for improving sleep, with certain essential oils having long been associated with relaxation and stress relief. **Lavender,**

for instance, is one of the most popular oils used to promote sleep. Studies have shown that the scent of lavender can slow the heart rate, reduce anxiety, and increase the amount of deep sleep, leading to a more restful night. You can use lavender essential oil in a variety of ways, from adding a few drops to a diffuser to creating a pillow spray that can be misted onto your sheets before bed.

**Chamomile** is another excellent essential oil for sleep, known for its calming and anti-anxiety properties. Chamomile has a gentle, soothing effect on the nervous system, helping to ease tension and prepare the mind for rest. Other scents like **sandalwood** and **cedarwood** have earthy, grounding aromas that promote calmness and can help reduce overthinking or anxious thoughts as you try to fall asleep.

Incorporating these oils into your bedtime routine can enhance the overall sleep experience. Diffusing oils into the air using a humidifier or essential oil diffuser is one of the simplest ways to enjoy their benefits.

Alternatively, adding a few drops of essential oil to your bath or massaging diluted oil onto your skin before bed can provide a more immersive, relaxing experience.

## Decluttering and Organizing for a Calm Mind

A cluttered, disorganized bedroom can create subconscious stress that interferes with your ability to relax. The mind often mirrors the environment, so if your space is messy, your thoughts may feel chaotic as well. **Decluttering your bedroom**is an important step in creating a space that encourages peace and tranquility. Start by clearing away any items that don't belong in the bedroom—piles of clothes, books, or work-related materials can create unnecessary distractions. Instead, aim to create a minimalist, serene environment that signals to your mind that this is a place for rest.

Organizing your space is not just about tidying up; it's about creating a layout that feels intentional and calming. Consider limiting the number of items on display and focusing on soft, soothing colors for your decor, such as cool blues, muted greens, or warm neutrals. Having a designated area for everything, like nightstand drawers or storage bins, helps keep clutter at bay and prevents you from feeling overwhelmed when you enter the room.

Even small touches, like making your bed each morning or setting out sleep essentials like your favorite book or a glass of water, can make your space feel more inviting. A clean, organized bedroom allows your mind to focus on rest rather than the chaos of the day, making it easier to slip into a peaceful night's sleep.

# Chapter 4: Mind-Body Techniques for Sleep

## Meditation and Mindfulness for Calming the Mind

In today's fast-paced world, one of the greatest obstacles to restful sleep is the inability to quiet the mind. Thoughts from the day can race through the head, making it difficult to wind down. This is where **meditation and mindfulness** come in as powerful tools for calming mental chatter and preparing the body for sleep. At its core, mindfulness is the practice of being present, fully engaging with the moment instead of letting the mind wander into the past or future. By focusing on the present, mindfulness can help reduce anxiety and stress—two major contributors to insomnia.

Meditation, specifically **mindfulness meditation**, involves sitting quietly and focusing on your breath or a specific word or phrase (a mantra), gently guiding your mind back when it wanders. Regular meditation practice has been shown to decrease activity in the brain's "default mode network," the part responsible for mind-wandering and self-referential thoughts, which can be overactive in people with insomnia. Even spending just 10 minutes a day practicing mindfulness can create a profound shift in your relationship with sleep.

When used at bedtime, mindfulness meditation can be transformative. Instead of lying in bed, allowing worries to grow, you can shift your attention to the sensations of the body and the rhythm of your breath, promoting a sense of peace. This practice encourages you to observe your thoughts without becoming entangled in them, ultimately allowing your mind to let go and settle into sleep.

## Breathing Exercises to Relax the Body

Breathing is one of the most immediate ways to signal to your body that it's time to relax. **Breathing exercises** can activate the body's parasympathetic nervous system, often referred to as the "rest and digest" system, which counteracts the "fight or flight" response that keeps you alert and anxious. By focusing on your breath, you can lower your heart rate, decrease blood pressure, and calm the mind.

One effective breathing technique for sleep is the **4-7-8 method**, which involves inhaling deeply through the nose for four seconds, holding the breath for seven seconds, and exhaling slowly for eight seconds. This practice slows down your breathing, which naturally relaxes the nervous system, easing tension in the body and helping to quiet the mind.

Another simple but effective technique is **diaphragmatic breathing**, also known as belly breathing. Instead of shallow breaths that only move your chest, belly breathing encourages deeper, fuller breaths that expand the diaphragm. This type of breathing promotes relaxation by maximizing oxygen flow and engaging the body's natural relaxation response.

Both techniques can be practiced while lying in bed, helping to shift your focus away from racing thoughts and toward the calming rhythm of your breath. With regular practice, these breathing exercises can become a reliable part of your nightly routine, signaling to your body that it's time to transition into sleep.

## Progressive Muscle Relaxation

While racing thoughts often keep us awake, **physical tension** in the body can be just as much of a hindrance to restful sleep. That's where **progressive muscle relaxation (PMR)** comes in—a technique designed to help you release tension in the body by focusing on and relaxing each muscle group, one at a time. The process involves tensing a muscle group as you inhale, holding for a few seconds, and then releasing the tension as you exhale.

This technique not only helps you identify where tension is stored in your body—whether it's in your shoulders, neck, or back—but also helps to physically release that tension, promoting a deep state of relaxation. The deliberate process of tensing and releasing muscles helps create a contrast that allows your body to feel progressively more at ease as you move through each muscle group.

You can start with your toes, slowly working your way up through the legs, abdomen, chest, arms, neck, and face. As each muscle group relaxes, you'll feel your entire body becoming heavier and more comfortable, making it easier to drift off into sleep. PMR is especially useful for those who experience stress-related muscle tension or have difficulty fully relaxing at bedtime.

## Visualization Techniques for Falling Asleep Faster

The mind is a powerful tool, and **visualization techniques** can use that power to help guide you into sleep. Visualization, also known as guided imagery, involves focusing on a mental image that brings about a sense of calm and relaxation. This technique works by redirecting your mind away from stressful or anxious thoughts and towards a serene, peaceful place, allowing your body to follow the mind's lead into rest.

One common visualization technique is to imagine a tranquil setting—a beach, a forest, or a favorite spot from your past. The more detailed your mental image, the more engaging it becomes for your mind, pulling you further away from the stressors of the day. As you visualize, focus on the sensations: the sound of waves, the feel of soft sand beneath your feet, or the warmth of the sun on your skin. The goal is to immerse yourself in this mental space so fully that your body begins to relax in response.

Another effective technique is **counting backwards** while pairing it with deep breaths. Imagine each number slowly drifting by, sinking further into a sense of calm as you exhale. This simple focus can distract your mind from anxiety-inducing thoughts and provide a meditative focus to help you fall asleep more quickly.

These visualization techniques, combined with other relaxation methods, can create a powerful wind-down routine that makes falling asleep an easier, more pleasant process.

# Chapter 5: The Power of Herbal Remedies

## Overview of Natural Herbs for Sleep

Natural herbs have been used for centuries to promote relaxation and improve sleep quality. Unlike synthetic medications, these herbal remedies work with the body's natural systems to ease anxiety, calm the mind, and prepare the body for rest. Some of the most effective herbs for sleep include valerian, passionflower, chamomile, and lemon balm.

Valerian is one of the most well-known herbal remedies for insomnia. It's commonly used as a sleep aid due to its ability to increase the levels of gamma-aminobutyric acid (GABA) in the brain. GABA is a neurotransmitter that reduces brain activity, helping you relax and fall asleep more easily. Valerian is particularly helpful for people who struggle with both falling asleep and staying asleep, as it has a calming effect without the grogginess associated with some medications.

Passionflower is another powerful herb that promotes sleep by calming the nervous system and reducing anxiety. Like valerian, it increases GABA levels in the brain, leading to a sense of tranquility. Passionflower is often recommended for people who experience restlessness, anxiety, or racing thoughts that keep them awake at night.

Chamomile is perhaps the most popular herbal sleep aid, often enjoyed as a tea before bed. Known for its mild sedative properties, chamomile is soothing both to the body and mind. It helps reduce inflammation, ease tension, and relieve mild insomnia symptoms, making it a gentle yet effective option for promoting better sleep.

Lemon balm is another herb that has been used for centuries to improve sleep and reduce anxiety. This herb has a mild sedative effect and is often combined with other calming herbs, such as valerian or chamomile, to create a more potent sleep remedy. It is especially effective for people who struggle with sleep due to stress or an overactive mind.

## How to Safely Use Herbal Supplements

While herbal remedies are generally safe for most people, it's important to use them responsibly, especially when incorporating them into a regular sleep routine. Herbal supplements should be treated with the same care and attention as any other form of treatment. Before starting any new herbal remedy, it's always a good idea to consult with a healthcare provider, particularly if you are taking medications or have existing health conditions, as some herbs can interact with medications or exacerbate certain medical issues.

When using herbal supplements, it's crucial to start with a low dose and monitor how your body reacts. Herbs like valerian or passionflower can have a sedative effect, and taking too much at once could lead to drowsiness the next day. Gradually increasing the dose based on your body's response can help you find the right balance for promoting sleep without unwanted side effects.

Another important consideration is timing. Herbal supplements should be taken around 30 to 60 minutes before bed to allow them time to take effect. Some herbs, like valerian, may need a few days or weeks of consistent use to fully develop their sleep-promoting properties. It's also essential to use high-quality supplements from reputable brands to ensure you are getting a pure and potent product.

For those who prefer not to use supplements, herbal teas or tinctures offer a gentler way to experience the benefits of sleep-promoting herbs. Teas and tinctures tend to have a milder effect, making them ideal for people who prefer a more subtle approach to improving their sleep quality.

## Preparing Herbal Teas and Tinctures for Nighttime Use

Herbal teas and tinctures are easy and effective ways to incorporate natural sleep remedies into your nightly routine. Herbal teas can provide a soothing ritual that signals to your body and mind that it's time to unwind. To prepare an herbal tea, simply steep dried herbs—such as chamomile, passionflower, or lemon balm—in hot water for 5 to 10 minutes. For a stronger effect, allow the herbs to steep for longer or use a larger quantity of herbs. Drinking the tea about 30 minutes before bed can help you relax and prepare for a restful night.

You can also combine several herbs to create a sleep blend tailored to your needs. For example, mixing chamomile with a small amount of valerian root can create a calming tea that eases both anxiety and insomnia. Adding a bit of honey or a slice of lemon can enhance the flavor while adding an extra element of comfort to your pre-sleep ritual.

Herbal tinctures are another convenient way to use natural sleep remedies. Tinctures are concentrated liquid extracts made by soaking herbs in alcohol or glycerin, which allows the active compounds to be preserved in a potent form. Tinctures are typically taken in small doses—just a few drops under the tongue or mixed with water or tea. Because they are more concentrated than teas, tinctures are especially helpful for people who need a stronger sleep aid or want a more portable option.

To make an herbal tincture at home, you can use dried or fresh herbs. Place the herbs in a glass jar and cover them with alcohol (such as vodka), making sure the herbs are fully submerged. Seal the jar and let the mixture sit for four to six weeks, shaking it occasionally. After this period, strain the liquid through a fine mesh or cheesecloth, and store the tincture in a dark glass bottle. You can take a few drops of the tincture before bed, either directly or mixed with water or tea, to promote relaxation and sleep.

By incorporating these herbal teas and tinctures into your nightly routine, you can create a calming, natural way to wind down and prepare your body for a good night's sleep. Whether you prefer a soothing cup of chamomile tea or a few drops of valerian tincture, these natural remedies offer gentle yet effective support for improving your sleep quality.

# Chapter 6: Aromatherapy and Essential Oils

## Understanding the Connection Between Scent and Relaxation

The sense of smell is deeply connected to our emotions and mood through the **olfactory system**, which directly communicates with the brain's limbic system—the part responsible for controlling emotions, memories, and even instinctual behaviors. This makes scent a powerful tool for influencing your state of mind. Certain aromas can trigger feelings of relaxation and calm, which is particularly beneficial when trying to ease into sleep. Smelling a soothing scent before bed can signal to your brain that it's time to wind down, helping to create a mental and emotional shift from the busyness of the day to a state of rest.

When you inhale a calming scent, it stimulates the olfactory nerves and activates a response in the brain, leading to reduced heart rate, lower blood pressure, and a decrease in stress hormones like cortisol. This process promotes a sense of tranquility, which is essential for falling asleep more easily. Aromatherapy, which uses natural plant extracts and essential oils, has been shown to help reduce anxiety, improve sleep quality, and even lengthen the duration of sleep.

## Best Essential Oils for Sleep

**Lavender** is one of the most well-known and researched essential oils for promoting relaxation and sleep. Its soothing floral aroma has been found to lower heart rate and blood pressure, both of which are essential for entering a relaxed state before sleep. Lavender's calming effects help ease tension and anxiety, making it easier to fall asleep and stay asleep through the night.

**Sandalwood** is another excellent choice for inducing relaxation. Its earthy, woody scent has a grounding effect that helps to quiet an overactive mind. Sandalwood is often used in meditation for its calming properties and is particularly beneficial for those whose insomnia is rooted in stress or anxiety.

**Roman chamomile** is a mild yet highly effective essential oil for promoting sleep. Its apple-like scent has a soothing effect on both the mind and body, and it is often used to reduce feelings of restlessness and agitation. Chamomile is gentle enough to be used by most people and can be especially helpful for those who experience mild insomnia or stress-induced sleeplessness.

**Cedarwood** has a warm, woody aroma that promotes emotional balance and calm. It helps stimulate the production of serotonin, which is then converted into melatonin, the body's natural sleep hormone. Cedarwood is ideal for creating a peaceful environment that encourages the mind to release the stresses of the day.

**Ylang-ylang**, with its sweet, floral scent, is known for its sedative properties. It works by reducing feelings of stress and anxiety, which can otherwise prevent sleep. Ylang-ylang is also thought to help lower heart rate and blood pressure, contributing to a more relaxed state before bed.

## How to Use Diffusers, Pillow Sprays, and Roll-Ons for Better Sleep

There are several simple and effective ways to incorporate essential oils into your bedtime routine. One of the most popular methods is using an **essential oil diffuser**, which disperses the oils into the air, filling the room with calming scents that can help you relax as you prepare for sleep. To use a diffuser, fill it with water and add a few drops of your chosen essential oil or blend of oils. Diffusers are a great way to gently introduce calming scents into your environment without being overpowering. For a restful night's sleep, try diffusing lavender or chamomile oil about 30 minutes before you go to bed, allowing the scent to fill the room as you settle in for the night.

If you prefer a more direct approach, **pillow sprays** offer a quick and easy way to enjoy the benefits of essential oils. Pillow sprays are essentially diluted essential oils that can be spritzed onto your pillow and bedding before you lie down. A spray with calming oils like lavender, sandalwood, or cedarwood can create an inviting and relaxing atmosphere as you drift off to sleep. The soft scent lingers on your pillow throughout the night, subtly promoting relaxation with each breath.

For those who want to enjoy the benefits of essential oils on the go or in a more concentrated form, **roll-ons** are a convenient option. Roll-ons are typically small bottles containing essential oils blended with a carrier oil, such as coconut or jojoba oil. You can apply them directly to pulse points, such as your wrists, temples, and the back of your neck. The warmth of your skin helps release the aroma, which can calm the mind and body. Applying lavender or Roman chamomile roll-ons just before bedtime can help induce sleep while creating a soothing nightly ritual.

Whether you choose to diffuse oils into the air, spritz them onto your pillow, or apply them directly to your skin, essential oils provide a natural and effective way to create a calming sleep environment. Incorporating aromatherapy into your bedtime routine can help shift your mindset and promote the deep relaxation necessary for a good night's sleep.

# Chapter 7: Sleep-Boosting Lifestyle Changes

## Importance of a Consistent Sleep Routine

Establishing a **consistent sleep routine** is one of the most powerful habits you can form to improve your overall sleep quality. Our bodies operate on a **circadian rhythm**, an internal clock that regulates when we feel awake and when we feel tired, based largely on a 24-hour cycle of light and dark. A regular sleep schedule helps align your internal clock with these natural cycles, making it easier for you to fall asleep and wake up at the same time each day.

When you go to bed and wake up at inconsistent times, it confuses this natural rhythm, making it harder to achieve deep, restful sleep. The body thrives on routine, and by sticking to a consistent sleep and wake schedule, even on weekends, you train your body to recognize when it's time to rest. Over time, your body will naturally adjust to this routine, reducing the likelihood of insomnia and improving overall sleep efficiency. A well-regulated sleep routine also enhances the quality of your sleep, ensuring you spend enough time in the deeper, more restorative stages of sleep.

Maintaining a consistent sleep routine isn't just about the hours spent in bed; it's also about setting up rituals that signal to your body that it's time to wind down. These bedtime habits, whether it's reading a book, taking a warm bath, or practicing relaxation exercises, act as cues that help transition your body and mind into a state of readiness for sleep.

### Reducing Screen Time Before Bed

In today's digital age, **screen time** is one of the most common factors interfering with our ability to fall asleep easily. The blue light emitted by phones, tablets, laptops, and televisions mimics daylight, which tricks the brain into thinking it's still daytime. This artificial light suppresses the production of **melatonin**, the hormone responsible for regulating your sleep-wake cycle, making it harder to feel sleepy when it's time to go to bed.

Limiting screen time in the **hour or two before bed** is crucial for improving sleep quality. Ideally, it's best to switch off screens entirely and engage in more relaxing, non-stimulating activities during this time, such as reading a book, listening to calming music, or practicing mindfulness. If eliminating screens altogether isn't feasible, there are ways to mitigate their impact. Many devices now offer **blue light filters** or "night mode" settings, which reduce the amount of blue light emitted, making it easier for your brain to transition into sleep mode.

In addition to the effects of blue light, the content consumed on screens can also be stimulating. Scrolling through social media, answering emails, or watching action-packed shows can keep the mind alert and engaged when it should be winding down. Reducing exposure to this kind of mental stimulation before bed can significantly improve the ease with which you fall asleep and stay asleep.

## Physical Activity and Its Connection to Sleep Quality

Regular **physical activity** is not only beneficial for overall health but also plays a significant role in enhancing sleep quality. Exercise helps regulate your body's energy levels throughout the day, leaving you physically tired and ready for sleep at night. Studies have consistently shown that individuals who engage in **moderate-intensity exercise**—such as walking, jogging, or cycling—tend to fall asleep faster, stay asleep longer, and experience deeper sleep than those who live a more sedentary lifestyle.

The connection between physical activity and sleep quality is linked to several factors. First, exercise helps to reduce **stress and anxiety**, two common culprits of insomnia. When you engage in physical activity, your body releases endorphins, which act as natural mood elevators, promoting feelings of relaxation and reducing tension. Regular exercise also helps regulate the body's internal temperature, which plays an important role in initiating and maintaining sleep. After a workout, your body temperature rises and then gradually falls, mimicking the natural temperature drop that occurs before sleep, signaling to your body that it's time to rest.

However, the **timing** of your physical activity is important. Engaging in vigorous exercise too close to bedtime can have the opposite effect, increasing your heart rate and stimulating your nervous system, making it harder to wind down. Aim to finish intense workouts at least three hours before bed to give your body ample time to relax.

## Benefits of Morning Sunlight for Regulating the Body's Natural Clock

Exposure to **morning sunlight** plays a crucial role in regulating your body's circadian rhythm, which dictates your sleep-wake cycle. Natural sunlight, particularly in the morning, helps synchronize your internal clock by signaling to your brain that it's time to be awake and alert. This early-morning exposure to light suppresses melatonin production, which naturally helps you feel more energized during the day and encourages the production of **serotonin**, the neurotransmitter associated with mood and well-being.

When you regularly expose yourself to morning sunlight, your circadian rhythm becomes more aligned with the natural cycles of day and night, making it easier for your body to know when it's time to wake up and when it's time to go to sleep. Sunlight exposure in the early part of the day can help you feel more awake and alert, while promoting melatonin production later in the evening when the light fades.

Morning sunlight also helps improve sleep by promoting **better energy levels** throughout the day. When your circadian rhythm is well-regulated, you experience more consistent energy during waking hours, reducing the need for naps or caffeine, which can otherwise interfere with your ability to fall asleep at night. Simply spending 20 to 30 minutes outside in natural sunlight within an hour of waking can have profound effects on your sleep cycle, helping you feel more alert during the day and more ready for sleep at night.

If you live in an area where natural sunlight is limited, particularly during winter months, **light therapy** lamps, which mimic natural daylight, can be a good substitute. These lamps are designed to help regulate your circadian rhythm when sunlight exposure is low, ensuring that your body's internal clock remains in sync with the environment.

By incorporating these habits into your daily routine—such as maintaining a consistent sleep schedule, reducing screen time before bed, engaging in regular physical activity, and soaking in morning sunlight—you can create the ideal conditions for better, more restorative sleep. These small changes can make a significant difference in how well you sleep and how refreshed you feel the next day.

# Chapter 8: Relaxing Evening Rituals

## How a Bedtime Routine Can Signal the Body to Wind Down

Just as your body responds to a consistent wake-up time, it also benefits greatly from a structured **bedtime routine** that signals when it's time to wind down for sleep. The human body thrives on patterns and cues, and establishing a regular routine before bed helps train your brain to recognize that it's time to transition from activity to rest. This creates a state of **anticipation for sleep**, helping to reduce stress and promote relaxation as bedtime approaches.

Your bedtime routine doesn't have to be complicated or time-consuming—it can be as simple as engaging in a series of calming activities that you enjoy. Over time, these actions become **triggers** for your body and mind to shift into a restful state. For example, dimming the lights, listening to soothing music, or sipping on a cup of herbal tea can signal to your brain that it's time to let go of the day's busyness and start preparing for sleep. The key is to keep your routine consistent each night, which reinforces the body's natural rhythm and helps to ease the transition into sleep.

## Gentle Yoga or Stretching Before Bed

Incorporating **gentle yoga or stretching** into your bedtime routine is an excellent way to relax both your body and mind before sleep. Yoga helps release physical tension that accumulates throughout the day, particularly in areas such as the neck, shoulders, and lower back. This tension can contribute to discomfort that makes it harder to fall asleep or stay asleep through the night. Gentle stretches, on the other hand, help to lengthen and relax tight muscles, promoting a sense of physical ease and calm.

Certain yoga poses, like **child's pose, legs up the wall,** or **cat-cow stretches**, are particularly effective in helping your body unwind before bed. These poses not only release physical tension but also encourage deep, steady breathing, which activates the body's parasympathetic nervous system, responsible for rest and digestion. By engaging in yoga or stretching, you can shift your body away from the "fight or flight" response associated with stress and into a more relaxed, restorative state.

Even a few minutes of stretching or yoga before bed can make a significant difference in how quickly you fall asleep and how deeply you rest. The rhythmic breathing and mindful movements help quiet the mind, making it easier to let go of the day's stressors and fully prepare for sleep.

## The Impact of Journaling and Gratitude Exercises on Sleep

**Journaling** and practicing **gratitude exercises** before bed are two highly effective techniques for clearing the mind and creating emotional calm before sleep. One of the most common causes of insomnia is an overactive mind, where thoughts from the day—worries, plans, or unresolved issues—race through your head as you try to fall asleep. Writing these thoughts down in a journal can help release them from your mind, making it easier to relax.

By journaling, you give yourself a space to process the events of the day, release pent-up emotions, and even solve problems that might be weighing on your mind. This can help reduce nighttime anxiety and provide a sense of closure to the day, allowing you to fall asleep with a clearer, calmer mind.

In addition to journaling, practicing **gratitude** before bed has been shown to improve sleep quality. Reflecting on the positive aspects of your day—no matter how small—can shift your focus away from stress and worry and toward feelings of contentment and peace. Writing down just a few things you're grateful for at the end of the day can foster a more positive mindset, helping you to feel more relaxed and at ease as you prepare for sleep. The act of gratitude also helps lower stress levels, which can be a key factor in reducing insomnia.

## Creating a Personal Wind-Down Routine That Works for You

While many common wind-down activities can be beneficial, the most important aspect of any bedtime routine is that it works for **you**. Everyone's body and mind respond differently to various techniques, so it's important to create a **personalized routine** that aligns with your preferences and lifestyle. Whether it's reading a book, practicing meditation, or enjoying a warm bath, the goal is to engage in activities that help you feel calm and relaxed.

To create your own wind-down routine, start by identifying activities that naturally help you relax. Experiment with different combinations of activities and see what works best for you. Some people may find that 10 minutes of mindfulness meditation followed by a cup of chamomile tea is enough to ease them into sleep, while others may benefit from incorporating stretching, aromatherapy, or quiet journaling into their routine. The key is consistency—choose activities that you can realistically incorporate into your nightly routine and stick with them.

Your wind-down routine should also avoid stimulating activities, such as checking emails or engaging in intense conversations, as these can keep the mind alert when it should be slowing down. The aim is to create a **sense of ritual**—a predictable, comforting sequence of actions that tells your body it's time to relax and prepare for sleep. Over time, your body will begin to associate these actions with rest, making it easier for you to fall asleep quickly and wake up feeling more refreshed.

By developing a bedtime routine that includes calming activities like gentle yoga, journaling, and gratitude exercises, you can create a powerful set of tools to ease the mind and body into a state of restfulness. A well-curated routine not only signals to your body that it's time to sleep but also enhances your overall sleep quality, making it easier to wake up refreshed and energized for the day ahead.

# Chapter 9: Alternative Therapies for Insomnia

## Acupuncture for Sleep

**Acupuncture** is an ancient Chinese practice that involves inserting thin needles into specific points on the body to promote balance and healing. Over the years, acupuncture has gained recognition in the West for its ability to alleviate a range of conditions, including insomnia. The practice is based on the idea that energy, or "qi," flows through the body along pathways known as meridians. When this energy is blocked or out of balance, it can lead to various issues, including poor sleep.

For those suffering from insomnia, acupuncture aims to restore this balance by targeting points associated with **calming the mind, reducing stress, and regulating sleep patterns**. Acupuncture may also stimulate the production of endorphins and other natural chemicals that promote relaxation. By addressing the underlying causes of sleep disruption, such as anxiety, chronic pain, or hormonal imbalances, acupuncture can help regulate the body's sleep-wake cycle, making it easier to fall asleep and stay asleep throughout the night.

Studies have shown that acupuncture can be particularly effective for people experiencing insomnia due to stress or anxiety, as it helps lower cortisol levels—the stress hormone—allowing the body to enter a more relaxed state. While acupuncture is generally safe, it's essential to consult with a qualified practitioner to ensure the treatment is tailored to your specific needs.

## Massage Therapy and Sleep Benefits

**Massage therapy** is another holistic approach that can significantly improve sleep quality by reducing stress, relieving tension, and promoting relaxation. Regular massage helps reduce the levels of **cortisol** while increasing **serotonin**, the neurotransmitter that helps regulate sleep. When serotonin levels rise, the body produces **melatonin**, the hormone that controls your sleep-wake cycle. This makes massage therapy particularly beneficial for those struggling with insomnia caused by stress, anxiety, or chronic pain.

In addition to its hormonal benefits, massage therapy promotes physical relaxation by releasing tension in muscles and joints. This can be especially helpful for individuals who suffer from conditions like **restless leg syndrome** or **chronic pain**, both of which can disrupt sleep. By loosening tight muscles and promoting circulation, massage therapy helps the body relax fully, making it easier to drift into sleep and stay asleep for longer.

Massage can be tailored to individual needs, with some focusing on deep tissue relaxation and others on gentle techniques designed to soothe the nervous system. Techniques such as **Swedish massage** or **reflexology** can be incorporated into a sleep-supportive routine, helping to release tension and create a sense of peace before bedtime. Even self-massage or the use of tools like foam rollers can provide similar benefits by promoting relaxation and reducing physical discomfort.

## Light Therapy and Melatonin Regulation

**Light therapy** is a non-invasive treatment that uses specific types of light to regulate your body's **circadian rhythm**—your internal clock that determines when you feel alert and when you feel tired. Exposure to light plays a crucial role in regulating **melatonin** production, a hormone that helps you fall asleep and wake up in sync with your natural rhythms. When your circadian rhythm is disrupted, either due to lifestyle habits or environmental factors like seasonal changes, your sleep patterns can become irregular.

In light therapy, patients are exposed to a **lightbox** or lamp that mimics natural sunlight, typically for 20 to 30 minutes a day, usually in the morning. This early exposure to bright light helps suppress melatonin during the day, promoting alertness, while encouraging the hormone's production in the evening, signaling to the body that it's time to wind down for sleep.

Light therapy is particularly helpful for individuals who suffer from **seasonal affective disorder (SAD)**, jet lag, or those who struggle with irregular sleep schedules due to shift work. By using light to regulate melatonin levels, you can help reset your internal clock, making it easier to fall asleep at the right time and wake up feeling refreshed. For those with insomnia related to light exposure, limiting artificial light in the evening and opting for light therapy in the morning can help reset your sleep cycle effectively.

## Sound Healing and Music for Deep Relaxation

**Sound healing** is an ancient practice that uses **vibrational frequencies** to promote deep relaxation and healing. In recent years, sound therapy has gained popularity for its ability to improve sleep quality by reducing stress, balancing energy, and helping the mind enter a state of **deep relaxation**. Instruments like **singing bowls, tuning forks, and gongs** are used to create sounds that resonate with the body's energy centers, helping to clear mental and physical blockages that may be preventing restful sleep.

**Music therapy** is another form of sound healing that has been widely studied for its benefits in promoting sleep. Listening to calming music, especially music with **slow tempos and soothing tones**, can slow down brainwave activity, reduce heart rate, and ease the mind into a restful state. Music therapy can be especially beneficial for people who have trouble turning off racing thoughts before bed, as it provides a focal point that helps distract from stress and anxiety.

Certain types of music, such as **classical music** or **ambient soundscapes**, have been shown to improve sleep quality by promoting relaxation and reducing sleep latency—the time it takes to fall asleep. Sounds like **white noise, rain, or ocean waves** can also mask disruptive environmental noises, creating a more peaceful atmosphere conducive to sleep.

For an added layer of relaxation, **binaural beats**—a type of sound wave therapy that uses two different frequencies in each ear to create a perceived third frequency—can help induce **theta brainwave activity**, which is associated with deep relaxation and meditation. Using these sounds as part of a bedtime routine can help quiet the mind and promote a deeper, more restful sleep.

Incorporating therapies such as acupuncture, massage, light, and sound healing into your sleep routine can significantly enhance relaxation and promote a deeper, more restorative sleep. Each of these methods offers unique benefits, allowing you to find the combination that works best for your body and lifestyle.

# Chapter 10: Natural Supplements for Insomnia Relief

## Overview of Natural Supplements Like Melatonin, Magnesium, etc.

**Natural supplements** can play a supportive role in helping to regulate sleep patterns and improve sleep quality without the harsh side effects associated with some prescription medications. Among the most commonly used natural sleep aids are **melatonin**, **magnesium**, **valerian root**, and **L-theanine**, each offering unique benefits for enhancing rest and relaxation.

**Melatonin** is a hormone naturally produced by the pineal gland that helps regulate the body's sleep-wake cycle. It's often referred to as the "sleep hormone" because of its role in signaling to the body when it's time to sleep. Melatonin levels naturally rise in the evening as the light fades, helping the body wind down for sleep, and fall again in the morning. For those who struggle with insomnia, irregular sleep patterns, or jet lag, taking a melatonin supplement can help regulate the body's internal clock and improve the quality of sleep.

**Magnesium** is another essential mineral that plays a critical role in promoting relaxation and reducing stress. Magnesium helps regulate the neurotransmitters in the brain that control sleep, and it also has a calming effect on the nervous system by activating the body's parasympathetic (rest and digest) response. Deficiency in magnesium is associated with increased stress, anxiety, and disrupted sleep patterns. For those who have difficulty falling asleep or staying asleep due to muscle tension or stress, magnesium supplements can help relax the body and promote a more restful sleep.

**Valerian root** is an herbal remedy commonly used to treat insomnia and anxiety. It is thought to increase GABA (gamma-aminobutyric acid) levels in the brain, a neurotransmitter that helps calm the nervous system and reduces overactivity, which can lead to better sleep quality. Valerian is often used as a natural alternative to sedative medications, and it is particularly effective for those who experience stress-related sleep issues.

**L-theanine**, an amino acid found in green tea, is another popular supplement for sleep. It works by promoting relaxation without causing drowsiness. L-theanine increases alpha brain waves, which are associated with a state of wakeful relaxation, making it easier to transition into sleep. For those who struggle with an overactive mind or stress before bed, L-theanine may help promote calmness and ease the body into sleep naturally.

## How to Incorporate Supplements Safely

While natural supplements can be highly beneficial, it's important to use them **safely** and **mindfully**. Each individual's body reacts differently to supplements, and what works for one person may not work for another. Before incorporating any new supplements into your routine, it's crucial to do your research and consult with a healthcare provider, especially if you are taking medications or have existing health conditions.

Start by using a **low dose** of any new supplement to assess how your body reacts to it. For example, with melatonin, a lower dose (0.5-1mg) may be sufficient to help regulate sleep without causing grogginess the next day. Many people mistakenly think that taking a higher dose will result in better sleep, but with supplements like melatonin, more isn't always better. A low dose is often enough to trigger the body's natural sleep process.

Another important consideration is **quality**. Look for reputable brands that have been third-party tested for purity and potency to ensure you're getting a high-quality product free from contaminants. Natural supplements are not regulated as strictly as prescription medications, so it's important to buy from trustworthy sources.

## Dosage and Timing Considerations

When taking natural sleep supplements, **timing** is key. For supplements like melatonin, it's best to take them about **30 minutes to one hour before bedtime** to give them time to take effect. Since melatonin works to regulate the body's internal clock, it's important to take it at the same time each night for consistency, particularly if you're using it to manage **jet lag** or **shift work** sleep issues. Taking melatonin too late at night may not give it enough time to promote sleep, and taking it too early may disrupt your natural rhythm.

**Magnesium** supplements, on the other hand, can be taken with your evening meal or about 30 minutes before bed. Since magnesium helps relax muscles and reduce tension, taking it close to bedtime ensures that your body can fully benefit from its calming effects. Magnesium is also available in various forms, such as **magnesium glycinate**, which is highly absorbable and known for its soothing properties without causing digestive discomfort.

For **valerian root** and **L-theanine**, it's important to start with a low dose and monitor how they affect you. Valerian can take a few weeks of consistent use to reach its full effect, while L-theanine generally works within

30-60 minutes of ingestion. Both supplements can be taken before bed as part of a calming routine.

It's essential to read the **recommended dosage** on each supplement label and not exceed the suggested amount. Too much of any supplement can have the opposite effect, potentially causing side effects like headaches, digestive discomfort, or grogginess.

## When to Consult with a Healthcare Professional

While natural supplements are generally safe for most people, there are certain instances where it's important to consult with a healthcare provider before starting a new supplement regimen. If you are **pregnant**, **breastfeeding**, or have **chronic health conditions**, such as **diabetes**, **high blood pressure**, or **thyroid disorders**, supplements like melatonin or valerian may interact with your condition or medications.

Those who are taking **prescription medications**—particularly **antidepressants**, **blood thinners**, or **blood pressure medication**—should be especially cautious. Some natural supplements can interact with these medications, potentially leading to adverse effects. For example, melatonin can interfere with blood-thinning medications, while valerian may enhance the sedative effects of certain drugs, causing drowsiness or slowed breathing.

In cases of **chronic insomnia** or **severe sleep disorders**, it's best to seek advice from a healthcare professional or sleep specialist to rule out any underlying medical conditions, such as **sleep apnea** or **restless leg syndrome**, which may require more targeted treatments.

By taking a thoughtful approach to supplements, starting with low doses, and consulting with a healthcare provider when necessary, you can safely incorporate natural remedies into your sleep routine and enjoy their full benefits for better rest and relaxation.

# Chapter 11: Managing Stress and Anxiety for Better Sleep

## Identifying Stress Triggers That Interfere with Sleep

One of the primary reasons people struggle to fall asleep or stay asleep is due to stress. The challenge, however, is that **stress** can stem from a variety of sources, and it affects everyone differently. To improve your sleep, it's important to first identify the specific **triggers** that might be interfering with your ability to relax and drift off at night. Stress triggers can be external, such as work-related pressures, financial concerns, or personal relationships, but they can also be internal, like perfectionism, self-criticism, or fear of the future.

**Work-related stress** is a common culprit, especially for those who find it difficult to switch off from their professional responsibilities. The never-ending to-do lists, tight deadlines, and pressures to perform can leave your mind racing at night. Similarly, **personal stressors** like family issues, relationship struggles, or health concerns can weigh heavily on the mind, preventing your brain from winding down.

Other more subtle stress triggers include **overstimulation**—from too much screen time, late-night news consumption, or even an overly packed schedule that leaves little time for relaxation. These seemingly small contributors can accumulate over time, creating a sense of constant alertness that makes it difficult to fully disengage and prepare for sleep.

The first step in addressing stress-related insomnia is to pay attention to **patterns**. What situations or thoughts tend to occupy your mind as you lie in bed? Are there recurring worries that surface each night? By identifying the specific sources of your stress, you can begin to address them directly and create strategies to manage them before they disrupt your sleep.

## Coping Techniques for Reducing Nighttime Anxiety

Once you've identified your stress triggers, the next step is to implement **coping techniques** to reduce **nighttime anxiety**. Anxiety can make it difficult to fall asleep, as your mind replays events from the day or fixates on upcoming concerns. The good news is that there are several strategies that can help quiet the mind and promote a sense of calm before bed.

One of the most effective coping techniques is **deep breathing**. Practicing slow, controlled breaths activates the body's **parasympathetic nervous system**, which calms the "fight or flight" response triggered by stress. Simple exercises, such as **box breathing** (inhale for four seconds, hold for four seconds, exhale for four seconds, and pause for four seconds), can help to lower your heart rate and relax your muscles.

Another powerful method is **progressive muscle relaxation**, where you systematically tense and then release different muscle groups in your body. This technique helps shift focus from anxious thoughts to physical sensations, allowing your body to relax and your mind to follow suit.

**Mindfulness meditation** is another coping tool that has been proven to reduce anxiety and improve sleep. By focusing on the present moment and letting go of worries about the past or future, mindfulness can help reduce the cycle of overthinking that often keeps people awake. Even a few minutes of mindful breathing or guided meditation before bed can create a sense of calm and help break the cycle of stress-induced insomnia.

## How Journaling or Cognitive Behavioral Therapy Can Help

**Journaling** is a simple yet highly effective tool for managing stress and improving sleep. Writing down your thoughts and feelings at the end of the day can help you process emotions, gain perspective, and release mental tension. Instead of letting worries build up in your mind, journaling allows you to **externalize** them, giving you a sense of control and closure. You don't need to write pages—simply jotting down what's on your mind, your to-do list for the next day, or even what went well today can be enough to clear your head for a more restful night.

One form of journaling that has been shown to be particularly helpful for sleep is **gratitude journaling**. By focusing on the positive aspects of your day, no matter how small, you shift your attention away from stressors and toward a more **positive mindset**, which can help promote relaxation and sleep.

For more persistent sleep struggles caused by anxiety, **Cognitive Behavioral Therapy for Insomnia (CBT-I)** can be a game-changer. CBT-I is a structured program that helps you identify and change **negative thought patterns** and behaviors that contribute to sleep difficulties. It focuses on reshaping your relationship with sleep by addressing misconceptions and breaking the cycle of anxiety around not sleeping. For example, CBT-I may help you challenge thoughts like "If I don't sleep tonight, I won't function tomorrow," replacing them with more balanced perspectives. This therapy can be particularly helpful for those with chronic insomnia related to stress and anxiety.

## Simple Ways to Unwind from a Stressful Day

The way you transition from your day to bedtime can make a significant difference in your ability to fall asleep peacefully. Developing a **wind-down routine** helps signal to your brain that it's time to shift gears from activity to rest. Here are some simple yet effective ways to unwind from a stressful day:

1. **Limit Stimulation**: Start by creating a buffer zone between your daily activities and bedtime. Reducing exposure to **stimulating content** like work emails, news, or intense television shows in the hour before bed helps prevent your mind from becoming overactive. Instead, focus on calming activities such as reading a book,

listening to calming music, or engaging in a creative hobby.

2.  **Take a Warm Bath or Shower**: A **warm bath** or shower can be a soothing way to relax both your body and mind. The warm water helps relieve muscle tension and promotes relaxation, while the drop in body temperature after the bath mimics the body's natural cool-down process that occurs before sleep, helping signal to your brain that it's time to wind down.

3.  **Practice Gentle Movement**: **Gentle yoga** or stretching can help release built-up tension in the body, especially in areas like the neck, shoulders, and lower back. These stretches encourage relaxation and help your body enter a restful state.

4.  **Create a Sleep-Friendly Environment**: Your environment plays a critical role in reducing stress and promoting sleep. Make sure your bedroom is a calm, restful space by keeping it cool, dark, and quiet. Aromatherapy, such as

using **lavender essential oil**, can enhance relaxation and prepare your mind for sleep.

5. **Engage in Relaxing Breathing or Meditation**: Deep breathing exercises, as mentioned earlier, can help lower stress levels and relax the body. You can also try **guided meditations** specifically designed for sleep, which use calming visuals and sounds to gently guide your mind into a relaxed state.

By incorporating these simple strategies into your evening routine, you can effectively reduce stress, quiet the mind, and prepare your body for a peaceful night's sleep.

# Conclusion

Finding restful sleep in the modern world can often feel like a challenge, but through the right combination of **holistic strategies**, a deep, rejuvenating sleep is entirely within reach. Throughout this book, we've explored a variety of natural approaches that address insomnia from multiple angles—whether it's adjusting your diet, creating a calming bedtime routine, practicing mindfulness, or incorporating natural remedies like herbal teas and essential oils. These strategies are designed to work with your body, gently guiding it back into balance and helping you rediscover the restful sleep that's essential for your overall well-being.

Each individual's sleep journey is unique, and that's why it's important to **experiment** with different approaches to find what works best for you. Perhaps you'll find that reducing screen time or adding some gentle yoga before bed helps you relax more easily, or maybe you'll benefit from incorporating magnesium into your evening routine. The key is to remain patient and open to trying different combinations of these techniques until you discover the ones that fit seamlessly into your life. Remember, the goal isn't to find a quick fix, but to develop habits that promote long-term, sustainable sleep health.

As you embark on this journey, know that reclaiming your sleep is not only possible but well within your grasp. By embracing a more **restful, balanced life**, you're not just improving the quality of your nights but enhancing your energy, focus, and mood during the day. Sleep is the foundation of everything we do, and when you make it a priority, the benefits extend far beyond the bedroom. Here's to a future filled with peaceful nights and revitalized mornings—where sleep comes naturally, and you awaken refreshed and ready to take on the day.